Breast Augmentation Surgery

All you need to know

Dr. Sheila Harrison

Disclaimer

This content serves to provide general information about the disease and aims to empower you to seek prompt medical assistance if necessary to prevent complications. It's essential to stress that this information is not a substitute for consulting a qualified physician. The field of medical science is continually evolving, and due to the dynamic nature of medical knowledge, we recommend seeking expert advice if you encounter any inconsistencies or intend to take action based on the information in this content. Never disregard professional medical guidance or delay treatment based on something you've read online, including this material, or from any other online source. Always remember that the internet cannot cure you; rather, healing comes through the guidance of medical professionals and the providence of God.

Table of Content

Disclaimer 1

Table of Content 2

Overview 4

Section 1 5

  What is Breast Augmentation Surgery? 5

  Common Reasons for Breast Augmentation
  Surgery 7

Section 2 11

  Types of Breast Augmentation 11

    Breast Implants Augmentation 11

    Fat Transfer Breast Augmentation 14

Section 3 15

  A Major Consideration before Opting for
  Breast Augmentation Surgery 15

    Types of Implants Used in Breast
    Augmentation Surgery 17

    Comparison of Silicone and Saline
    Implants 18

    Breastfeeding And Breast Augmentation
    Surgery Issues 19

Section 4 21

  Risk Factors for Breast Augmentation
  Surgery 21

Section 5 23

The Breast Augmentation Surgery
Procedure Process   23
    Procedure Details   24
        At the Consultation for Breast
        Augmentation   24
        At the Preparation Level for Breast
        Augmentation Surgery   26
        Establishing a Home Recovery Area   28
        Surgical Procedure level for or On the
        day of the surgery level   29
Section 6   32
Post-operative Recovery process of a
Breast Augmentation Surgery   32
    How Long Do Breast Implants Typically
    Last?   33
    Life after Breast Augmentation   34

Overview

Breast augmentation is a common cosmetic surgery procedure that involves the use of breast implants or fat transfer to increase the size and shape of your breasts. There are various types of breast implants and surgical methods available, so consult with your surgeon to determine which is ideal for you.

The most common type of cosmetic surgery is breast augmentation. In the United States, around 300,000 people have breast augmentation surgery each year.

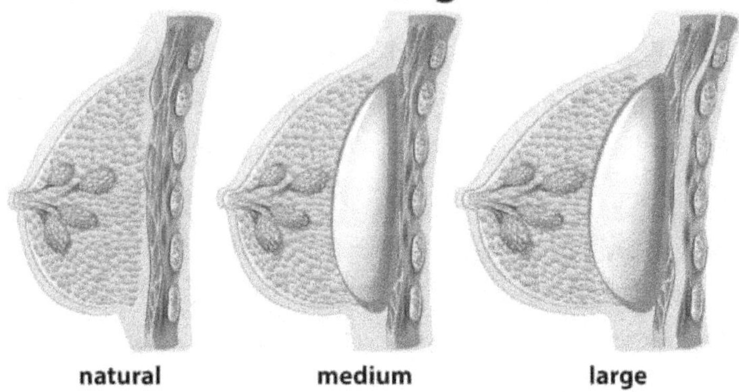

Section 1

What is Breast Augmentation Surgery?

Breast Augmentation Surgery vs Breast Augmentation Mammoplasty is a surgical surgery that enlarges the breasts. Typically, this is accomplished through the use of implants or fat transfer. Breast augmentation surgery entails inserting breast implants beneath the breast tissue or the chest muscles. This surgery is primarily performed for cosmetic reasons. However, the procedure may also be performed for reconstructive purposes, such as after a mastectomy for breast cancer.

Breast augmentation is not the same thing as breast lift surgery. While breast augmentation surgery can improve the size and form of the breasts, increasing the patient's self-confidence, breast lift surgery does not modify the size of the breasts appreciably. Breast lift surgery can provide the illusion of bigger breasts by raising sagging breasts and repositioning the nipples. A breast lift is frequently performed in conjunction with a breast augmentation.

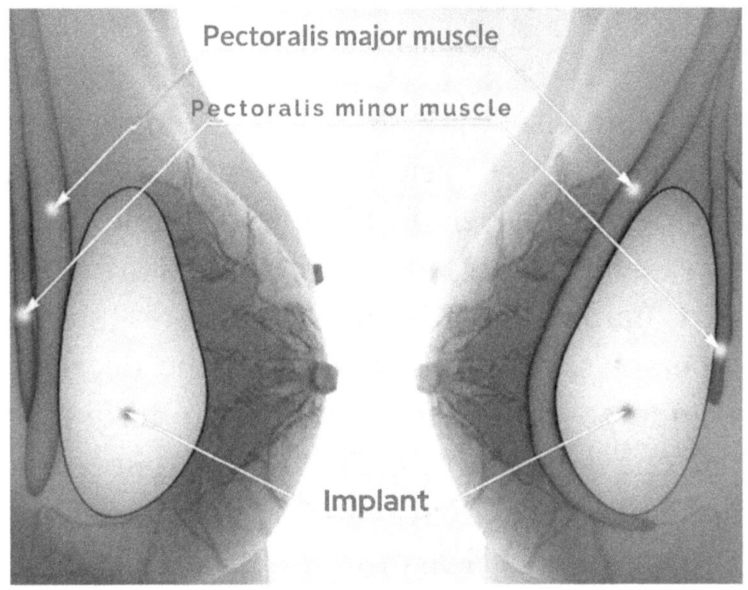

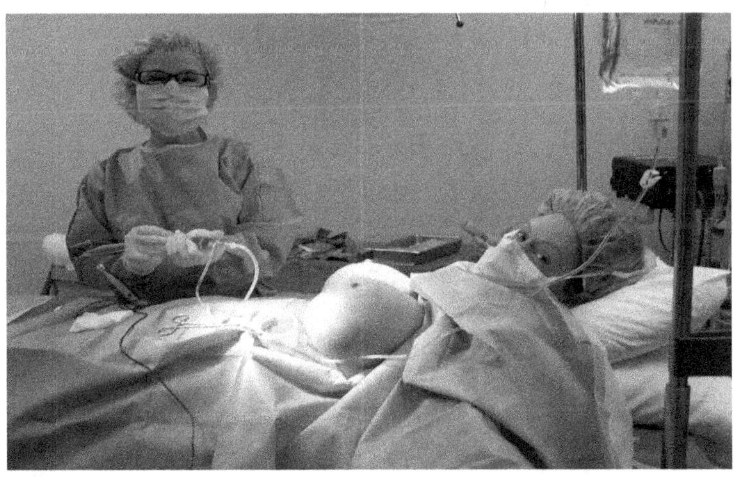

Common Reasons for Breast Augmentation Surgery

Individuals undergo breast augmentation surgery for a variety of reasons, which vary widely from person to person. Some of these reasons are personal, while others are medical in nature. You should be aware that each person's path is unique, and the decision to undergo breast augmentation is frequently a deeply personal one. The following are some of the most prevalent reasons why people choose to get this surgical procedure:

- **Personal happiness and self-confidence:** Many people choose breast augmentation surgery to improve their personal satisfaction and self-confidence. People frequently feel that perceived physical improvement can lead to increased self-esteem and overall happiness.

- **Restoration after mastectomy:** Many women prefer to have mastectomy after a mastectomy, which is a surgical operation that surgeons frequently do to treat or prevent breast cancer. In some circumstances, breast augmentation surgery is performed not just for cosmetic reasons, but also to restore a sense of femininity that may have been impacted by the mastectomy.

- **Cosmetic Balance:** The size of certain women's breasts may appear disproportionate to their body structure. Breast augmentation may be used by some people to develop a more balanced figure, resulting in a better body image.

- **Breast Asymmetry Can Be rectified:** Breast asymmetry, which is extremely prevalent, can be rectified by breast augmentation. While some asymmetry is typical, for some people, the discrepancy is more evident. In such circumstances, breast augmentation may be performed to balance the size of the breasts.

- **Breast reconstruction following pregnancy and breastfeeding:** Pregnancy and breastfeeding can drastically alter the size and form of a woman's breasts. Breasts may sag or lose volume as a result of post-pregnancy changes. As a result, for some people, the purpose for breast augmentation surgery may be to restore the breasts to their pre-pregnancy appearance, as culturally, people often equate it with youthful energy and femininity.

- **As a male-to-female surgical process:** Strong evidence suggests that breast augmentation is important in the MTF transition process. Many transgender women want breast augmentation as part of male-to-female (MTF) transition surgery, believing that it will aid in their transformation. This surgical treatment, also known as augmentation mammoplasty, involves enlarging the breasts by implanting saline or silicone-filled prostheses behind the chest muscles or breast tissues.

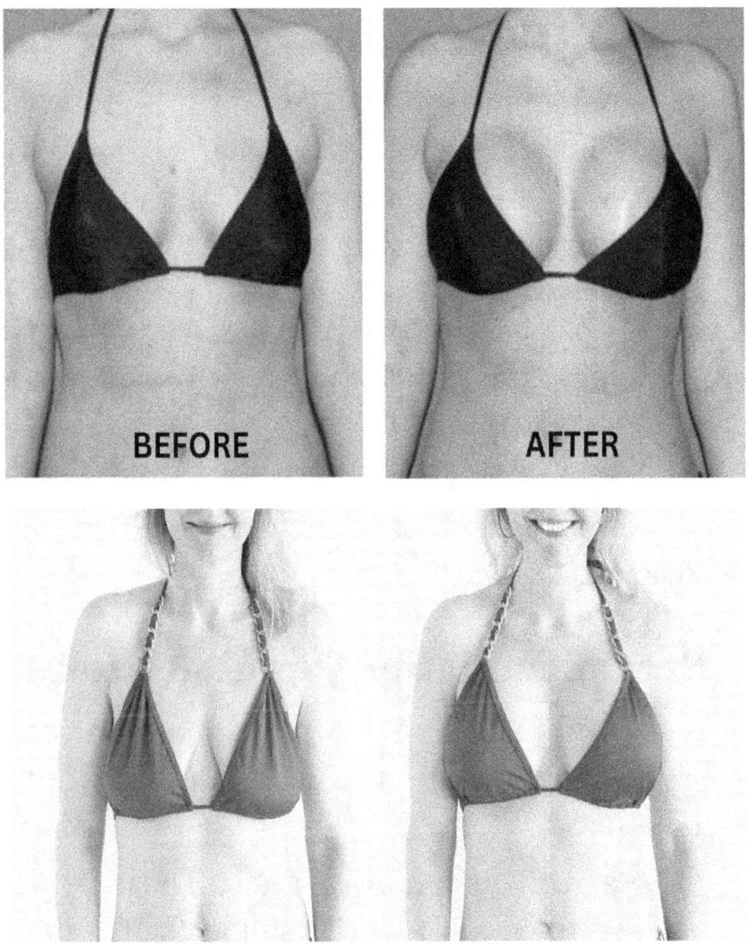

Section 2

Types of Breast Augmentation

Breast augmentation is classified into two types: breast implants and fat transfer augmentation. Within those two categories, there are other alternatives depending on how you want your breasts to look and feel. particular breast implants are only FDA-approved for particular ages. Before deciding on breast augmentation, it is critical to thoroughly research and understand the benefits and disadvantages of each option, as well as consult with a board-certified plastic surgeon.

Breast Implants Augmentation

Breast implants are the most common type of breast augmentation. Breast implant options include:

- **Saline breast implants:** These implants are filled with sterile saline (salt water). If the implant were to break inside your breast, your body will absorb the saline and naturally get rid of it.

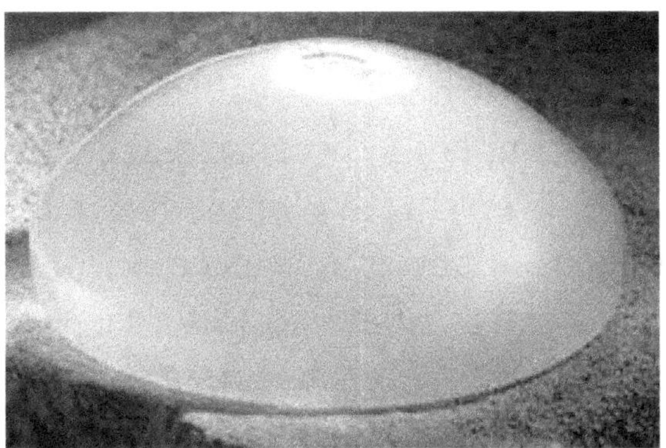

- **Structured saline breast implants:** These implants are filled with sterile saline (salt water) and have an inner structure that helps the implant feel more natural.

- **Silicone breast implants:** These implants are made of silicone gel. If the implant were to break, the gel could stay within its shell or leak into your breast.

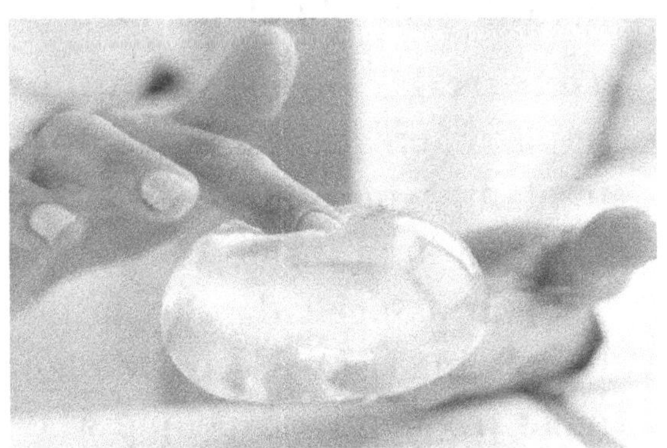

- **Form-stable breast implants:** These implants are often called gummy bear breast implants because they keep their shape even in the implant shell breaks. They are made of a thicker silicone gel and are firmer than traditional implants. Form-stable breast implants require a longer surgery incision in your skin.

- **Round breast implants:** These implants usually make breasts look fuller. Since the implants are round all over, they don't typically change the look of your breast if they rotate out of place.

- **Smooth breast implants:** These implants feel the softest of all the different kinds of implants. Smooth breast implants usually make breast movement look more natural than other implants.

- **Textured breast implants:** These implants create scar tissue to adhere to the implant, which makes them less likely to move around inside of your breast. Breast implant-associated anaplastic large cell lymphoma (BIA-ALCL), though rare, occurs most frequently in people who have breast implants with textured surfaces.

Fat Transfer Breast Augmentation

In a fat transfer breast augmentation, your surgeon will use liposuction to take fat from another area of your body and then inject that fat into your breasts. This type of augmentation is usually for people who want a relatively small increase in their breast size. In most cases, your surgeon will take fat tissue from one of the following areas:

- Your belly.
- Your flanks (the sides and lower back of your abdomen).
- Your back.
- Your thighs.

Breast Augmentation with Fat Transfer

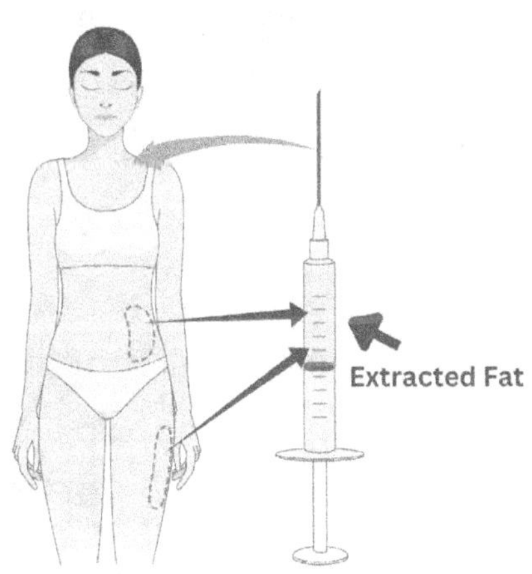

Section 3

A Major Consideration before Opting for Breast Augmentation Surgery

The two major considerations before opting for a breast augmentation surgery are the size of the implant and the type of the implant.

- An individual must make the correct choice when considering breast augmentation surgery in terms of both implant size and shape. The choice of implant size and shape must be a result of a balanced deliberation that takes into account not only aesthetic aspirations but also the individual's body structure and health conditions.

- The second most important consideration is the type of implant for increasing the breast size. The type of implant chosen affects the longevity, maintenance and aftereffects of the surgery. It is necessary to understand the types of implants, discuss this with your surgeon and decide accordingly.

While breast augmentation can provide instant satisfaction, it is important to take into account the long-term implications. You must have regular check-ups with your surgeon to ensure the integrity of the implants and to address any concerns or complications that may arise.

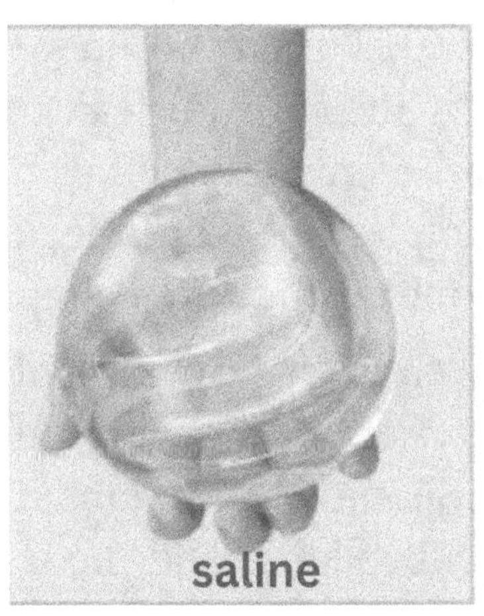

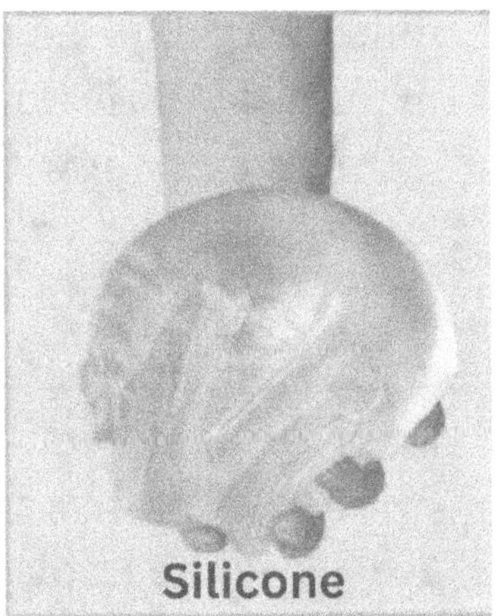

Types of Implants Used in Breast Augmentation Surgery

Breast implants are typically filled with saline or silicone gel. It is worth remembering that the specific needs and aesthetic goals of the patient influence the selection of implants for the surgery. The choice of implants typically falls within two principal categories.

One of the types of implants used in breast augmentation surgeries is silicone implants. It is filled with silicone gel and is often chosen for its natural feel. However, if the implant leaks, the gel may remain within the implant shell or may escape into the breast implant pocket. A leaking implant filled with silicone gel may not collapse.

Saline implants are another type of implant in breast augmentation surgery. They are filled with sterile salt water. Should the implant shell leak, a saline implant will collapse and the body starts absorbing saline and naturally expelling it.

Comparison of Silicone and Saline Implants

The choice between silicone and saline implants, which is often one of the most important decisions before a breast augmentation surgery, is not one that you make in haste. A comprehensive understanding of the pros and cons associated with each type of implant is crucial. The preferred type of implant varies greatly among individuals, depending primarily on their personal preferences, their health history, and their aesthetic goals.

Implant Type	Pros	Cons
Saline	Safety, adjustability, smaller incision	Feels less natural
Silicone	Feels natural, less risk of rippling	Rupture may not be noticeable without an MRI scan

Breastfeeding And Breast Augmentation Surgery Issues

While breastfeeding is possible for females there may be some complications that arise as a result of breast augmentation surgery.

The type of surgery performed plays a significant role in determining whether breastfeeding will be possible or not. Specific information regarding different types of surgeries and their potential impacts on breastfeeding are below:

Type of Surgery	Potential Impact on Breastfeeding
Incision made under the breast (Inframammary)	Most likely will not impact breastfeeding
Incision made around the areola (Periareolar)	Potential risk to milk ducts, which may affect breastfeeding

Incision made in the armpit (Transaxillary)	Less likely to impact breastfeeding as there are no incisions on the breast itself

For trans-women and non-binary people, induced lactation using adjuvant hormone therapy has been studied with some success. However, it is still not a common medical practice.

Section 4
Risk Factors for Breast Augmentation Surgery

Within the realm of breast augmentation surgery, a topic that frequently comes up is the potential for breast implants to rupture or leak. This is indeed a possibility, albeit one that is not overly common.

Implant rupture, also frequently referred to as an implant leak, is a situation in which the breast implant's outer shell experiences a tear or hole. When that occurs, the gel or saline solution within the implant can begin to leak into the surrounding tissues.

- **Saline Implant Rupture:** When a saline implant ruptures, the body will typically absorb the saline solution, thereby causing the implant to deflate. This deflation is usually noticeable within a matter of hours or a few days at most. Given that the body is able to absorb the saline solution naturally, doctors do not usually consider it harmful. However, the deflation of the implant will necessitate a surgical procedure to replace it.

- **Silicone Implant Rupture:** Unlike saline implants, a rupture in a silicone implant may not be immediately apparent. This is due to the fact that silicone gel tends to remain within the tissues surrounding the implant, rather than being quickly absorbed by the body. This situation, often referred to as a 'silent rupture', can go unnoticed for an extended period of time.

Although researchers generally do not consider the silicone gel as harmful to the body, the FDA recommends regular monitoring of silicone implants through MRI or ultrasound imaging to check for potential ruptures.

Section 5

The Breast Augmentation Surgery Procedure Process

Doctors usually perform breast augmentation surgery as an outpatient procedure under general anesthesia. It is essential to note that breast augmentation surgery is a complex procedure that requires skilled medical intervention. After they administer anesthesia, the surgeon carefully makes incisions in inconspicuous areas to minimize visible scarring. They may make these incisions in the natural crease of the breast, the axilla (armpit), or around the areola. This depends on the patient's anatomy, the type of implant, and the degree of enlargement desired by the patient. Therefore, if you are about to undergo the procedure, you should adequately prepare yourself.

Following the incision, the surgeon inserts the breast implant in a pocket, either:

- Under the pectoral muscle (a submuscular placement), or

- Directly behind the breast tissue, over the pectoral muscle (a submammary/ subglandular placement).

Once the surgeon properly positions the implant, they stitch up the incisions. Sometimes, they may use tape or skin adhesive to close the skin. Over time, incision lines will fade significantly.

Procedure Details

At the Consultation for Breast Augmentation

Before you undergo breast augmentation, you'll meet with your plastic surgeon. You should prepare for this consultation by thinking about what you want to change about your breasts. Remember, you're not seeking perfection, but improvement. Also, be sure that you're in good mental and physical health, overall, and that you have realistic expectations.

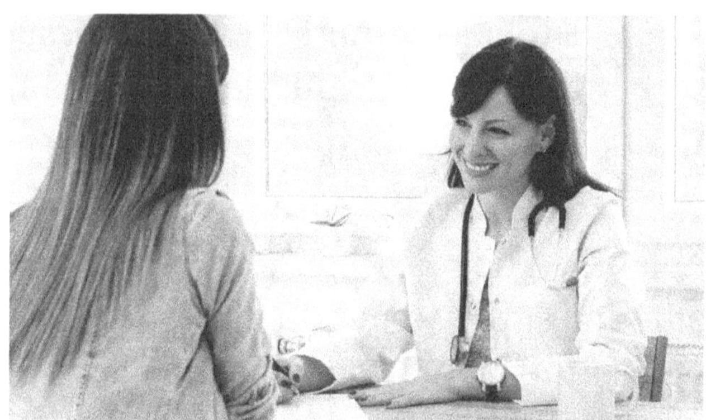

Your surgeon will ask you detailed questions about your medical history, including:

- What medications you are taking.
- What allergies you may have.
- Your smoking history.
- Prior surgeries.
- Any previous issues you've had with your breasts, including lumps, previous mammograms and any family history of breast issues.

It may be helpful to ask your surgeon the following questions during your breast augmentation consultation:

- Are you certified by the American Board of Plastic Surgery?

- How many years have you been a plastic surgeon?

- How often do you perform breast augmentations?

- Can I see some of the before-and-after pictures from the augmentation surgeries you've performed?

- Should I get breast implants or have a fat transfer?

- What are the pros and cons of the different types of breast implants?

- Will I be able to breastfeed after breast augmentation?

- What are the risks of my type of augmentation surgery?

- What will happen if I'm not satisfied with the results of my augmentation?

At the Preparation Level for Breast Augmentation Surgery

In preparation for your breast augmentation surgery, your surgeon may have you:

- Get a blood test.
- Take certain medications or adjust your current medications.
- Stop smoking.
- Avoid certain foods or beverages.
- Avoid taking aspirin and certain anti-inflammatory drugs, since they can increase bleeding.
- Stop using recreational drugs.

It's crucial to follow any instructions that your surgeon gives you before your surgery. Following their instructions will help the surgery go more smoothly and will help you heal properly.

You should arrange for someone to drive you home after your surgery and also have someone stay with you the first night at least. You will need to take at least three days off from work, so plan accordingly. If you have a labor-intensive job, you will likely need to take off at least three weeks of work.

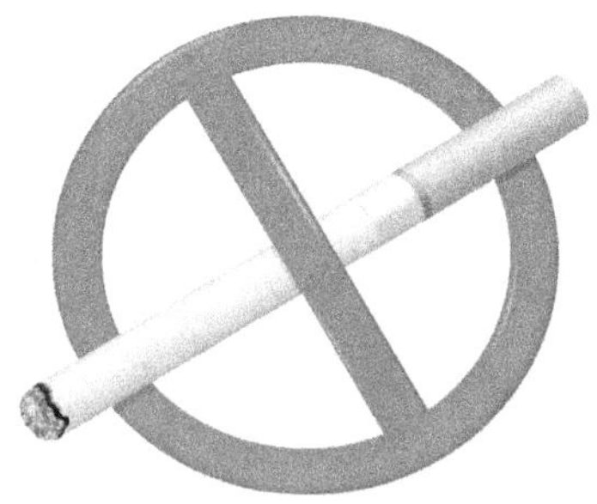

Establishing a Home Recovery Area

Before you undergo breast augmentation surgery, you should set up an area in your home for recovery. Make sure you have:

- Pain medication prescribed by your surgeon and/or acetaminophen (Tylenol®).

- Ointment or cream for incision sites (if recommended by your surgeon).

- Clean gauze to cover the incision sites.

- Plenty of loose, comfortable, button-down blouses or shirts.

Surgical Procedure level for or On the day of the surgery level

There are many steps involved in breast augmentation surgery. Here's an explanation of the steps.

Anesthesia

Your surgeon will perform the surgery while you are under general anesthesia (you'll go to sleep) or through IV sedation. You and your surgeon will determine this together.

The Incision

Breast augmentation can be performed in one of several ways.

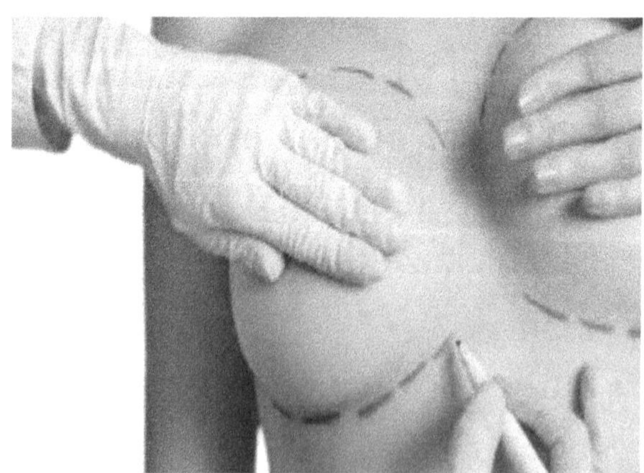

Your surgeon can perform the procedure:

- Via the crease under your breast (known as the inframammary fold).

- Along the edge of your areola (known as the periareolar incision).

- Via your armpit (known as a transaxillary approach).

Your surgeon will discuss these possible methods with you before your surgery, and together you will determine which approach best suits your needs.

Implant Insertion

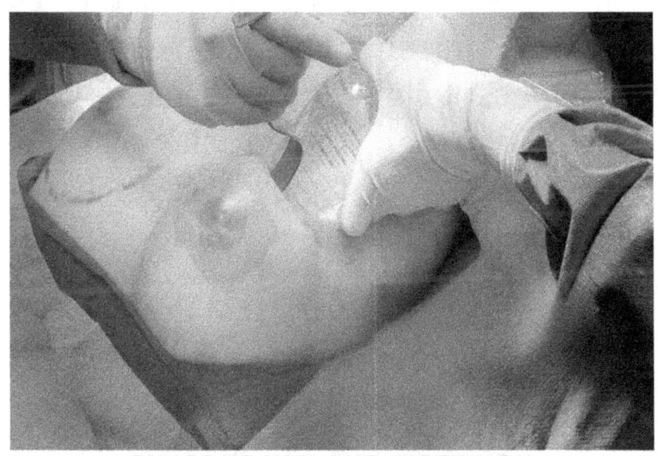

SILICONE INPLANT INSERTION

There are two different ways for your surgeon to insert the implant: under your breast tissue and in front of your muscle or behind your breast muscle (pectoral muscle).

The placement of the implants depends on a few factors, including the type of implant you choose and how much you're increasing the size of your breasts. You can discuss the benefits of each method with your surgeon and make that decision together.

Closing the Incision

After your surgeon places your implants, they will stitch the incision sites together to close them. Your surgeon may also use drainage tubes. You must follow your surgeon's follow-up care instructions for the incision site. Your breasts will be covered with a gauze bandage and you may be sent home wearing a surgical bra.

Section 6

Post-operative Recovery process of a Breast Augmentation Surgery

While the immediate recovery period following breast augmentation surgery may vary, doctors generally discharge the patients on the same day as the surgery. You should have someone accompany them home and stay with them for at least the first night following the surgery. You will recover from the breast augmentation surgery and will be able to return to work and normal activities within a few days. However, you must avoid strenuous activities, particularly those that increase blood pressure, for several weeks.

How Long Do Breast Implants Typically Last?

The lifespan of breast implants, which is often a critical consideration for those contemplating breast augmentation surgery, can vary considerably. It is contingent upon a multitude of factors. Hence, it is not possible to give a precise, universal timeline. However, breast implants are generally not lifetime devices. One may need to replace them at some point.

Though multiple factors influence implant longevity, manufacturers of breast implants usually provide a 'product life expectancy' which is commonly around ten years. However, you should consider it more like a rule of thumb rather than a definitive endpoint. A multitude of women have implants that last significantly longer than this. Despite this, you must know that complications such as implant rupture or capsular contracture could necessitate earlier replacement.

Life after Breast Augmentation

Right after your breast augmentation surgery, a healthcare provider will take you to a room for observation while you wake up from the surgery. You'll be able to leave the hospital once you're stable enough. This usually takes around an hour.

Before you leave, your surgeon will give you specific instructions for your breast augmentation surgery recovery and schedule a follow-up appointment. Your surgeon will give you a prescription for medication to control pain, if necessary. If you have drainage tubes, your surgeon will tell you when to return to have those removed, as well as instructions as to when to remove the gauze bandages.

Your surgeon will probably remove your stitches in about one week. You should not do any heavy lifting for at least four weeks. If you are physically active in sports, it may take up to six weeks before you can return to those activities.